Burnout

When Your Brain Just Quits

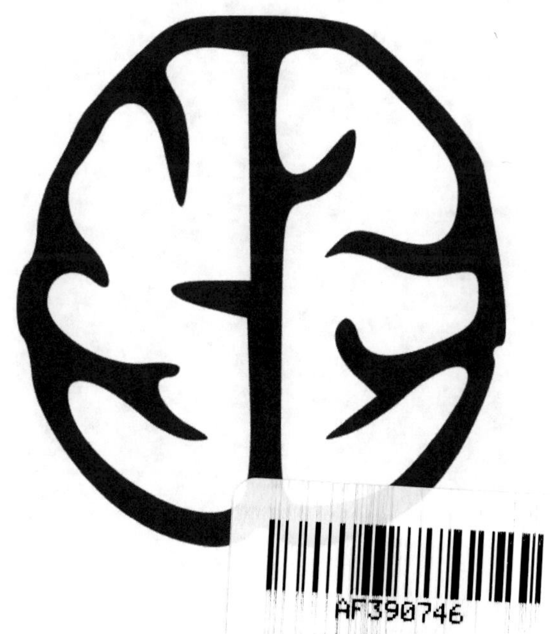

Noé GRATON

ISBN 978-2-9582777-0-3 (french, paperback, 2022)
ISBN 978-2-9582777-1-0 (french, Kindle, 2022)
ISBN 978-2-9582777-2-7 (french, Kobo, 2022)
ISBN 978-2-9582777-6-5 (english, paperback, 2023)
ISBN 978-2-9582777-7-2 (english, Kindle, 2023)

Acknowledgments

I want to thank all my loved ones for supporting me during this ordeal – my wife, my daughters, my sister and my in-laws. Being surrounded by loved ones is indispensable for healing. Even if they suffered from my situation, they never stopped trying to help get me out of the rut I was in.

I also want to thank my friend Christophe, who called me almost every day to see how I was and to joke around. He and I have passed through the business world with similar hardships and it has been a good example for me to see him launch a new career.

I thank as well my former colleagues, who regularly stopped by for drinks during my sick leave. Maintaining these ties of friendship allowed me to reconstruct real, authentic reference points that are now the foundation of my new life.

I thank my former neighbors for courageously coming to my aid and for all the goodwill they have always shown, both now and in times past.

I thank my attending physician and my psychologist for having handled my care so effectively during this long recovery. I commend their energy and their professionalism. They are all the more deserving of recognition since burnout is still not very well known or treated in the medical world.

Table of Contents

1 The day my body gave up on me

Saturday, January 4, 2020. Christmas vacation is drawing to a close. In two days, it will be back to work. These two weeks of rest had done us a world of good. We were able to enjoy some quality family time, slow down a bit, clear our minds, get some fresh air.

It's 1 p.m. We have just eaten and cleared the table. I am making a coffee for myself and plan to go sit in front of the TV. My wife, seated in front of me, is looking at me with a relaxed expression. But then suddenly, she looks worried. "Is everything OK? You're making a strange face."

"I've been feeling totally worn out lately. I think that I've really managed to unwind during this vacation, I really needed it."

For several days, I've been having a sort of load bearing down on my chest, a really strange sensation. It's not just a feeling of heaviness, it's a real physical pain, not very strong, but piercing. Something that I hadn't felt since childhood: this sort of contraction of the diaphragm and the rib cage that occurs when you feel a major sadness and sob heavily for a long time.

I hope that I'm not going to suffer a burnout. I need to hold on for several months more in order to get past this complicated period: the construction of our house, finally being able to move in, and finish the large project that I'm responsible for at work. During my check-up last June, the doctor at my work warned me, "Mr. Graton, you are in stage 3 of burnout. You need to slow down immediately, otherwise you are at major risk. If you break down, it will be very, very complicated."

Slow down. For a long time, I've felt that I've been doing everything I can in order to slow down. For several months, I've been forcing myself to do no more than the bare minimum: oversee the construction of our house and keep the project team running at work. We're not going to meet our business targets this year, but oh well, it's not the end of the world!

The doctor's warnings keep running through my head: "Force yourself to say no, don't take up any commitment...it doesn't all depend on you...you always have the choice!"

Nice words, but the reality is that whatever you do, there is always a minimum to deal with, and when this minimum is still too burdensome, you're stuck. I recall some details from this discussion. I told him," Imagine if you were a truck driver: if you feel tired and overwhelmed, you're nevertheless not going to say to your boss, 'Sorry, today I'm staying at the depot, I'll just wash the trucks and handle the tire pressure.' You were hired to drive a truck, and so the minimum is to do that, even if you go slower. In my case, I was hired to manage a team and spearhead projects, that's my minimum, I can't get out of it. Thus, I'm either fit for work and have to keep performing my duties, or I am not fit, and I need to take medical leave. I don't see a middle point between the two."

After my check-up, I had a discussion with my boss to explain the situation to him. We were both aware of the burden weighing on me and we had decided to take draconian measures: stop all my business trips until further notice and add resources to help my team. Nevertheless, the pressure was still there. Days that were already too short, spent solving other people's problems, unending requests, interruptions, a cumbersome and ineffective organization that relied on completely unsuitable tools and procedures, with no clear mechanism to improve the situation.

So that's it, I'm suffering a breakdown? No, it's not possible, I'm coming out of vacation, I'm relaxed, I haven't felt so peaceful in a long time. But this pain in my chest is not going away. What if my heart is giving out? Too much pressure, my heart is used up and now I'm going to have a heart attack? I share some of my worries with my wife. It's true that I've been feeling weak since this morning. I need to listen to my body, I have to see a doctor. Tough luck, we're in a medical desert, my primary doctor is fifty kilometers away and it's impossible to get an appointment in this region on a Saturday, at short notice.

In the end, we make up our minds: I ask my wife to drive me to St. Marcellin Hospital, which has an emergency consultation service that doesn't require an appointment. Maybe it's nothing, but if it's serious, it would be stupid to sit around and do nothing. Too bad for this last weekend of vacation, we'll have to spend part of it in a waiting room.

After filling in our daughters on the situation, we set off. But after two hundred meters, I tell my wife, "Wait, stop, I don't feel well." I feel like I could pass out at any moment. "If I pass out in the car, you won't be able to do anything, you'll have to resuscitate me on the side of the road. That would be the worst situation imaginable, take me back to the house." We turn around, but the few meters separating us from the house seem endless. My head and my chest feel like they're caught in a vise, my vision clouds up, my legs feel like jelly. I rally my last strength to drag myself out of the car and cross the distance that separates me from the couch to collapse there. It's not getting any better. My wife and my daughters bustle around me: they take my pulse, they touch my forehead. A sharp pain starts to spread through my left arm. There's no doubt now, I'm having a heart attack! In spite of the pain and my state of weakness, I remain perfectly conscious. My reflexes as a former first-aid worker start to resurface. I calmly explain the situation to my wife and my daughters, I give them instructions to follow: "Girls, you are going to ring at the neighbor's door and tell them that I'm feeling faint. Ask them to go get a defibrillator from the city hall and to get ready to use it. Honey, I'm probably going to lose consciousness in the next few minutes. You'll need to lay me down on the ground right away. Then, you'll check my pulse and my breathing. When that's done, call the fire department. If you can't feel a pulse, you'll have to start CPR while waiting for the defibrillator. Remember, you locate the midpoint of the sternum and press on the bottom part, firmly and deeply, one compression per second and two mouth-to-mouth breaths for every five compressions."

There I am, stretched out on the floor of the living room. The pain in my chest keeps getting sharper. I start shaking violently, I feel my limbs going numb: first a tingling, then a complete paralysis of my arms and legs, I can't move anymore. I have difficulty breathing, I'm out of breath, I'm swallowing huge gulps of air but it has no oxygen, my brain is shutting down, I can't see, everything is happening as if I no longer have any blood flow, I'm leaving this world. In a state of semi-consciousness, I see people flurrying about me. My wife is holding my legs up in the air to allow oxygen to flow to my brain. One neighbor is taking my pulse, while another massages my upper body to stimulate me. Hang in there, the firefighters are arriving! The defibrillator is ready, but you still have a pulse." I no longer have any sense of time. I think of my wife and my daughters, I see in their face that they're terrified but so courageous. What could be more horrible than to inflict such an experience on the ones you love! I try to speak to them, so that they see that I'm still there. I can't feel my body at all anymore, I don't understand why. I'm still conscious, but my body is no longer there. I only find that it's endless, I don't know how long I'm going to hold on.

A good forty minutes go by in this situation, but I no longer have any sense of time. My arms and legs are all tingly again. It hurts, like when you fall asleep on top of your arm and the blood starts to flow back in. My sight seems to be clearing up. I'm shaking violently, but I feel like my body is fighting, maybe I will pull through in the end. Somebody is standing over me. "Sir, do you hear me? I'm the doctor of the emergency response unit." The firefighters are here, the paramedics as well. The room is full of people moving about. I find myself quickly covered in sensors and devices. The crisis is over, I can feel my limbs again. My chest still feels tight and in pain, but you could say that I'm coming back to life little by little. It was a close call!

The doctor examines me all over for a while, asking me questions. She finally concludes, "Mr. Graton, I can't find anything abnormal. Your heart is fine, your pulse and blood pressure are perfect. The firefighters are going to take you to the emergency room for more tests."

After an ambulance ride, I spend the rest of the day at the emergency room under observation. In the evening, the ER doctor come to see me and explains that I'm totally fine. "Is it possible that I'm suffering from burnout?" I explain my fears to him, in light of the warning given to me by my work doctor. "It's entirely possible, you'll see about that with your primary care doctor, but for us, burnout is not a medical event. For my part, what I can observe is that you had a panic attack."

Unbelievable! I stumble back out on my wife's arm, with a piece of paper in my hands – the emergency room report, which concludes: "Chest pain from anxiety."

Well, there you go! See if you can make heads or tails out of that!

2   The medical ordeal

Who would have thought that a panic attack could be so intense? I spend Sunday dozing on the couch. I don't understand what's happening to me. This panic attack really knocked me out, I have no strength left. It's impossible for me to stay standing. I quickly realize that it's almost impossible for me to hold a conversation: I can't find my words, I need time to understand what they're saying to me and after a few minutes, I completely zone out, with my brain overloaded. I watch a TV program without understanding what it's about, it goes too fast for me. My memory is not great either. You surely must have found yourself in the middle of a room before, asking yourself, "What was it I was looking for?" Well, for me, that's a permanent state of being. I constantly lose my train of thought and can no longer concentrate on anything.

I seriously begin to consider that I'm burned out. That's it, I am. These are the problems that they had been warning me about for months. But to be clear, what is a burnout exactly? What happened and what is going to happen? I feel like my brain is overcooked, I'm only the shadow of my former self now.

Monday comes. I notify my employer about what is going on with me and try to get an appointment with a general practitioner. All the "normal" doctors only take appointments several days in advance and are not taking on new patients. Since we've lived in this region, I've never managed to find a new primary care doctor. Fortunately, I haven't needed to see the doctor very often, but on those rare occasions, I've only found space with a sort of crotchety old doctor that everybody avoids. In the neighborhood, everybody has a story to tell about him: "He almost killed me twice," "He gave me the wrong prescription," "He didn't even see that I had chickenpox," "He dislocated my shoulder while handling me," etc. In short, a world champion. But there was no choice, I had to see a doctor, if only in order to go on sick leave: it would be impossible to go to work when I can't even stand on my own two feet and I could barely speak!

So, there was our world champion, analyzing the emergency room report. Upon reading the conclusion, his face lights up. "Everything's OK, Mr. Graton, it's not your heart, nothing to worry about!" "Yes, OK. I understood that but it would appear that in any case I'm really burned out, no? How is it that I have no more energy? I can't even remain standing!" I go off in my explanations, I tell him everything I've experienced, the warning from the work doctor, and all the symptoms that I've noticed so far. I sense that he's annoyed, and in the end he's forced to examine me, begrudgingly. Then he finishes by saying, "If I understand correctly, Mr. Graton, you are one of those professionals who put pressure on themselves on their own. You've brought this on yourself, you well knew that you needed to slow down. So, tomorrow, go back to work, talk to your boss and tell him that he needs to reduce your workload." I am so flabbergasted that I cannot even raise a peep in protest.

I leave the doctor's office in tears, I don't understand this situation at all. My wife picks me up and hoists me into the car. I have a hard time explaining to her what I've just gone through. I don't know anymore what's going on with me. Have I gone crazy? All the doctors tell me that I'm fine. But why is it then that my body doesn't respond anymore, why is it so hard for me to put one foot in front of the other? My wife looks at me and says, "I see you and I believe you. Have no doubt, what you feel is real. I know you perfectly and I can assure you that you're not well. So we'll find another doctor and we'll get you treatment." I can never thank enough this marvelous woman who has always understood me and supported me.

Two years after these events, I realize to what extent the situation could have become critical if she hadn't been there to support me. If I had listened to that doctor and gone back to work, who knows what state I would be in today. With the benefit of hindsight, I know what burnout is and that's exactly the challenge of this illness: to understand what it involves. That's the longest and most difficult part, since no one will do it for you.

As I arrived back home, a miracle occurred. Yes, a miracle, I have to say. Without it, I might be in a psychiatric hospital by now. As I passed through the front gate, our neighbor was there, tinkering on who-knows-what with his car. He came up to me to ask for an update, and the words he spoke radically altered my destiny.

"You know Noé, what has just happed to you is a huge burnout. I know, you can believe me, I suffered the same thing five years ago." He told me about his misfortune, its symptoms, his long road to recovery. Finally, I began to understand! I wasn't crazy or the only person in the world with mysterious symptoms. Now, I knew: burnout really does exist, it's a real illness, not just feeling run down because you've pushed yourself too hard and are tired! Even if many people in the medical field are unfamiliar with it, today, I can affirm loud and clear that burnout is a full-fledged medical affliction with its wounds and its consequences!

I left again, carrying in my pocket the address of the doctor and the psychologist that allowed my neighbor to recover. "Call them and say that I sent you. They will take you seriously. You'll see, it's a long road. At first, you'll have to understand what has happened to you, that can take years, and only then will you know what to do. Maybe you will never completely heal from certain things, like me, who's permanently retired due to disability. But you will emerge stronger in everything else." This enigmatic prophecy, reassuring and yet worrying at the same time, marked the beginning of my long recovery...If you ever can really recover from a burnout!

3   The mechanism of burnout

Wow, as someone who rarely set foot inside a psychologist's office, I had a totally distorted image of them. I thought that – like you see in the movies – they were there to listen to the laments of fragile people who needed a friendly ear. But no, they are really useful. There are even some situations where they are completely indispensable. My psychologist treated me for a whole year and today I can clearly see that I would have never recovered without her help. Keep in mind, it's not nothing: she allowed me to understand what was going on in my head. And given the state my head was in at the time, that was no easy feat!

The first thing that I became aware of was that burnout is an illness that is at the same time widespread and yet unrecognized. Sure, the media harps on about how "It's the malady of our age, blablabla..." But so long as we fail to understand what this illness really entails, we don't realize the number of people who suffer from it. In fact, a large part of them don't even have to chance to put a name on it. In this way, we hear about whatshisname who "went on social security" because he didn't feel like working, Mrs. So-and-So who can't get off anti-depressants, besides "it would do her some good to get off her ass, life's not a bed of roses." And this "good-for-nothing" who ended up getting fired from his job because, all of a sudden, he could no longer put up with aggravation, told everybody off, and no longer wanted to be involved in the life of the business. Does that sound familiar to you? Behind each of these situations, there is perhaps an undiagnosed and untreated burnout that has seriously worsened.

According to my psychologist, it appears that there are as many types of burnout as there are victims. And that's exactly why the medical field has trouble integrating this illness into its classification system. The causes, the development and the symptoms of this illness can vary radically from one person to another. But the physiological phenomenon is always the same and we can summarize it as being "when your brain just quits."

Yes, yes, that seems crazy, but this phrase really sums it up. Burnout happens when the brain, for one reason or another, decides to no longer give orders to the rest of the body. A sort of paralysis, but less radical and less final.

Every individual possesses what psychologists call an "inner self," which constitutes the core of our intellect. It defines our functioning as an individual and the totality of the deep values that we embody. At once the result of the innate and the acquired, it's a real jewel, fashioned by millions of years of the evolution of the human race, by our education and by our experience. In most people, this inner self is noble and pure, it's what enables us to love and makes us capable of life in community, with respect for others and our environment.

At the same time, the circumstances of life lead us to play roles all the time. Some of these roles are natural and sincere. Most of the time, we manage to play these roles in harmony with our inner self: the role of spouse, parent, citizen...

But our modern lifestyle also means that we play roles that are totally out of sync with our inner self: the role of manager, team leader, employee, employer, or simply work colleague. The working world rarely creates conditions that are conducive to people behaving in an authentic way, to showing themselves in their true light. You need to be tough and protect yourself in order to be able to give and receive orders without bowing and scraping, to be effective and hard-nosed to hit the targets set for us. We construct an armor around ourselves and format our behavior and our speech to what the company expects of us. How can we be ourselves in such conditions, when our brain has been programmed at its deepest levels to function in a different way?

There's a name for feeling like you're somebody you're not: alienation. If there's one word to remember, it's that one. After one year of therapy, the verdict was clear: in my case, alienation was the main underlying cause of my burnout. Stress and mental load contributed to this, of course, but they were just aggravating factors.

When we're alienated, our mind has to carry out a risky and exhausting balancing act to manage the discrepancy between our external body and our inner self: it ensures that our words and our deeds are in keeping with the requirements of the role that is expected of us, while remaining aware that we are doing it in disharmony with who we really are.

When this alienation is too large and difficult for too long, the brain no longer has the strength to fight. However, our mind can't yield entirely to the requirements of this role and conform to it, that would be the end, the inner self would cease to exist. So in order to protect itself, it adopts an amazing defense mechanism: it abandons our body, it stops giving it orders. Not in order to let it die, but to force it to molt, to change its skin.

If we could hear our inner self speaking at this moment, it would say, "Sorry, I'm heading out. I'm leaving this body that doesn't belong to me anymore."

From that point on, the procession of symptoms becomes logical. All the functions that have to do with directing the body are affected:

- The action of the muscles: you feel an extreme, constant tiredness, even though you were in good shape.

- Motor coordination: you become clumsy, uncoordinated.

- Speech: you are at a loss for word, you can't manage to form sentences.

- Understanding: you hear without understanding, people have to repeat the message over and over again.

- Memory: you forget everything, people's names, you lose track of what you were doing.

- Concentration: it's impossible to read for more than 2 minutes at a time, every minor task becomes an ordeal.

- Some people seem to suffer from hormonal problems, mood issues, weight gain, etc.

- Finally, the symptom that is the hardest to pinpoint and heal: a sort of "psychological allergy" to everything that is the cause of this alienation. You become hypersensitive to manipulation and bad faith, to lying and malice. It's really striking to see to what extent the victims of burnout become sincere and authentic people, probably too direct, to tell the truth, likely to offend others sometimes. As someone who was always discreet and empathetic, I would take a thousand precautions with my words in order to never cause conflict or tension. But nowadays, I surprise myself by often saying things in a blunt, direct way. I always do so with the best of intentions, but I am no longer capable of "pretending" or being hypocritical. I know that my brain will no longer allow itself to be alienated.

It's difficult to grasp the extent of these symptoms without having lived them. They are all overwhelming and destabilizing. When my new attending physician began to take over my treatment, the first thing he asked me to do was to engage in as much physical exercise as possible in order to provoke my brain to reconnect with my body. Obviously, it was impossible to practice intense sports, but I needed to walk at least one hour per day, calmly, at my own pace. Well, during the first weeks, it was totally impossible for me to walk for more than five minutes. The desire was there and I enjoyed it, but my body just didn't respond. I would set off at a moderate, but determined pace, and after a couple dozen meters, my strides became shorter, slower, I had no more strength, I was completely out of breath and my legs started to give way. I was thus forced to turn back or otherwise find myself in distress.

At the beginning, you feel something that resembles muscle fatigue, but without the soreness. It feels as if your muscles had melted and had much less strength. Then as you heal, after several months, motor coordination comes back, you recover your normal dexterity and muscle strength....That is, the strength of someone who hasn't worked out in several months. So nothing special. At this stage, you might be tempted to think that you're back in business, you just need to start an exercise program and everything will go back to the way it was. Unfortunately, it doesn't work like that, because there remains a deeper sort of fatigue, without a doubt of a purely psychological nature. The will and the motivation are there, but that energy is still lacking, that sacred flame that makes you get up out of your chair and act without even thinking. In fact, you are obliged to do everything forcing yourself in a conscious manner. Burnout really gives you the sensation of having burned up that reserve of vital energy that allows us to act naturally in daily life.

I think this was the hardest thing to grasp during my recovery. With hindsight, it's become clearer. Now when I have to try to explain it, I like to use the example of those popular stories where an ordinary person finds the strength to lift up their car because their child is trapped underneath. The key is to understand that the physical capacity of our body is one thing, but the intensity with which we activate it is something else! Even high-level athletes are largely in agreement on this point: they all say that physical training is important, but in order to achieve real feats of athleticism, your mindset also has to be up to it.

I'm not enough of an expert at medicine or biology to explain why, but there is probably a mechanism that modulates the intensity of the signal that the brain sends to the muscles. Is it the intensity of the electrical current sent through the nerves? The density of a chemical exchange? I'm not sure. But it all works as if we had a reservoir of this vital kinetic energy: the reservoir fills up when sincere desires and motivations emerge, while its level falls when we force ourselves to act against our will. Thus, when alienation becomes omnipresent and when no sincere motivation appears to resupply the reservoir, it ends up emptying out completely. All our energy has been used up – thus giving us the very apt term "burnout."

So it seems obvious that we can only restore this energy reserve once our mind is totally at peace with the underlying causes that have driven us to burnout in the first place. In my case, it took at least a year and a half, during which I felt like I was in the body of an old man. I had to force myself for the most minor movements of daily life, even though my willpower and motivation were still intact.

I emphasize this symptom of bodily fatigue, because it is very disconcerting and all the more difficult to convey to those around you.

So take note, it's not just an act. When someone is burned out and stays splayed on their couch, it's not out of laziness, it's because their body is really not responding anymore.

And if they stay there without talking to you, with a distraught look, it's not that they're sulking, it's just that they don't understand what you're saying and can't formulate a sentence to answer you.

Now, let's debunk a false idea that has wide currency: "He's depressed." No! Burnout has nothing to do with nervous depression, these are totally distinct illnesses. But it is true that a misunderstood and mismanaged burnout can easily lead to an immense despair that triggers depression. My case illustrates well this distinction, since during my burnout I never felt any low spirits. I always maintained intact my will to live and bring my projects to fruition. But you can bet that the situation would have been different if I hadn't been so well supported by my family and my friends, or if I had been late in getting diagnosed and receiving treatment.

4 Personal misfortunes

At the start of my therapy, my psychologist asked me to draw up a list of all my misfortunes. I was really annoyed. I've never considered myself as someone unfortunate. I even have a lot of admiration for people who have to face dramatic hardships, like the death of a loved one or a serious illness and who despite it all, still have that spark that pushes them to appreciate every instant with a smile. On the other hand, I personally have never had any real personal drama, I've been fortunate to be well supported and to benefit from a certain material comfort. In short, I've always felt fortunate, and I wrongly believed that burnout always affects the unfortunate.

Thus, my psychologist asked me to write up the list of things that upset me, either things from daily life or the occasional hassles that I've had to face. And at that point, there were so many that it took weeks to catalogue them.

Between 2001 and 2012, we lived in a small village in Isère, to the north of Grenoble. From our first year of employment, my wife and I decided to invest our salaries in the construction of a house. Mortgages were much more affordable back then and, by tightening our belts a little, we could become owners of a small house measuring 90 m2 in a rural area with good infrastructure. It's there that we built our cozy little nest and raised our two daughters. It wasn't all easy, we both worked hard, but we peacefully advanced towards an improvement in our quality of life.

The plot that neighbored our own was occupied by a former event hall that had been reconverted into a municipal hall, where several events that enlivened the village took place: the old people's lottery, the conscripts' banquet, the movie club, the Christmas market, the theater club, the PTA refreshment stand, the yard sale, etc. All this helped create a nice atmosphere in the village, which we were happy to take part in. Then there was a change of town council and the new team decided that it was prudent to restore this building to its original function as an event hall. They began renting it out for next to nothing, first to residents of the village for the rare family event, such as weddings, baptisms, and birthdays. Then, in the space of several months, the event hall ended up being reserved several days per week by people who came from all over the department, drawn by the pleasant setting and the unbeatable price.

It goes without saying that our life radically changed. We spent sleepless nights weekend after weekend, stressed out by the sound system of these dance parties. Many times I would start my work week on Monday at 3 a.m. to catch the train or plane, not having had a wink of sleep the night before. By day, the situation was hardly any better. The cars coming and going and the games of pétanque in the parking lot gave us no respite, our life became a living hell.

Naturally, I engaged in talks with the mayor, asserting the totally illegal character of the situation, since the operation of sites "receiving the public and playing amplified music" are subject to very strict requirements. The mayor was aware of the inconvenience but claimed that he could do nothing, since bringing the hall up to standard would have been too expensive, and he could not get out of his obligations to the people renting the hall, as it was now booked solid for the next two years! Out of desperation, I finally filed a complaint with the police, but no tangible progress was made during the term of office of this unscrupulous mayor. The next municipal team improved the situation by installing a sound limiter that automatically cut off the power supply whenever the partiers were making too much noise. It was a bit more livable, but the underlying problem remained, to the extent that we seriously began to think about moving.

In terms of work, I was more and more weighed down. I've always loved my profession of product design engineer, but I was undergoing a growing pressure, to the extent that every day I told myself that it would be materially impossible for me to work in this industry for my entire career. It would be the death of me before I reached retirement age. Thus, the idea began to take root in me of branching out on my own and starting my own business. My profession and my experience allowed me to imagine a wealth of possibility, and I might as well work in a field that excited me.

And as it happens, when I reached the venerable age of 40 years old, my loved ones gave me a great gift by financing a training course in lutherie: two intensive weeks during which I learned to manufacture violins from A to Z. As an amateur violinist since my earliest childhood, lutherie had always fascinated me and this training course was the start of a real passion that I dreamed of making my profession.

But a career change is a step that needs to be carefully prepared. I would need a site that could be converted into a workshop, which our current house could not offer. Thus, if we needed to move into a house that would lend itself to such a purpose, we would have to do it before my career change, while my salary was still compatible with a new mortgage. After such a career change as I was planning, my income would inevitably take a nosedive, at least temporarily, and no banker would then speak to us. It would be necessary to do things in the right order.

One fine day, while my daughters were on an outing to their grandparents' place, my wife and I decided to go around to try to discover a new spot that would be a good place to live. In our mountainous region, there were only really two rural areas that were accessible enough and that had more or less decent real estate prices: Trième and the Chambarans. We had a large relief map hanging on the wall of the office. Our first step involved identifying the sunny little villages on the south-facing hillsides of the Chambarans.

We spent the day driving through the villages, with the map in one hand and the real estate listings in the other. In the middle of the afternoon, the small road we were following wound up through the forest and all of a sudden, a clearing opened up before us at the top of a hill. The horizon was massive, you could see 360 degrees all round. A small town was nestled into this backdrop, which we decided to explore. As soon as we got out of the car, we were engulfed in a soothing silence, only interrupted by the cries of buzzards circling above our heads. We spent the rest of the afternoon wandering through the village and on the hiking trails in the vicinity. We were enchanted.

A sign that read "lot for sale" caught our attention, but the location had poor sun exposure and was hard to reach. All the same, we decided to call the number of the real estate agent displayed on the sign. "I have two lots for sale in this village, would you like to visit them?" One of these lots was apparently the miserable place where we were at, but we were eager to discover the second one.

In just a few minutes, the real estate agent arrived and started giving us his spiel. We hurried through our visit to this first lot, then the realtor led us down a gravelly path that hugged the hillside and opened up onto a large field with a gentle slope and facing south, with a panorama to take your breath away of the Vercors range, the Drôme region and the Chambaran hills. "Here it is," he said. The look that passed between me and my wife at that moment will remain etched in our memories. We were astounded. We had struggled so much to find the site for our first house. We had had to make concessions, in particular the proximity of that damn event hall. And here we had stumbled onto a hidden gem. An opportunity that only comes about once in a lifetime!

In short, as you can imagine, in that moment our destiny changed dramatically. We knew that a difficult transition was in the offing, but it was worth it.

Events moved quickly: the purchase of this unbelievable lot, the sale of our current house and the search for rental housing near our future building site. Happenstance and the lack of supply in this area led us to rent an absolute dump: a small house from the 1960s, poorly insulated, unsanitary, run down, squeezed into a very steep plot and made completely inaccessible due to brambles. But we didn't care, we were happy and "it wouldn't be for a long time."

Unfortunately, it started to be one hassle after the other. The project seemed to be jinxed – it was a real voodoo curse!

First off, the general contractor in charge of managing the construction of our future house told us that he was going out of business, only a short time after he had filed our application for a building permit and had extracted from us an exorbitant sum. The blueprints were magnificent, an absolute dream, everything met our expectations. The application had been signed by the architect, filed with the Urban Planning Department, and was soon approved in due form. Everything started without a hitch, but all of a sudden, we found ourselves stopped dead in our tracks.

But no matter, we had to move forward at all costs. Our builder found a new general contractor, who quickly proved to be a totally incompetent layabout. The preparation of the price estimate was endless, we were forced to look for and contact the companies ourselves in order to move things forward, but without any result. The quotes did not arrive and when we finally managed to put a price on the construction, we had to face the facts: it was more than double our original budget! Oh, the architect drafted a beautiful house for us, we couldn't not be bowled over! But she just neglected to respect our budget.

There would be no way we could pay a new architect to modify the blueprints, we needed to save money for the rest of the project. So I had to redesign the house entirely myself! Guided by the builder in order to reduce the costs, everywhere it was possible and through some serious brainwork, I ultimately managed to put together a more realistic set of blueprints and to file for an amended permit.

Construction began two months later – one year late – in the rain and the mud. One tradesman followed the other, each more incompetent and negligent than the other. Each of them went from small slip-ups to consequences that were more or less disastrous. The new general contractor was

AWOL in spite of our constant pleading, to the point that I was forced to take days off every week in order to keep a close eye on the work site and try to catch any slip-up as it occurred. The culmination of this was when we discovered that the house was 70 cm too high and exceeded the maximum height authorized by the planning regulations. I realized after the fact that our general contractor had taken the initiative to build the walls higher than we planned without notifying us!

Fortunately, the builder assumed responsibility and got everything in progress to solve the problem. The roof was already in place with its tiles, and it was impossible to dismantle it. It was thus necessary to prop it up in order to keep it in the air while we made the walls shorter. Then, we brought the roof down, gradually loosening the props. A massive operation. After this ordeal, I still had to file a third application for an amended permit in order to bring the roof's final height into compliance, which involved another additional three months of delay.

One Saturday morning, somebody rang at the door: "Hello, I'm a court bailiff and I'm here to serve a summons." Our future neighbor out back, upset at having a new house in her field of vision, had decided to file an action against our building permit, past the deadline and based on a totally bogus and indefensible pretext. Luckily, I'm a perfectionist and our application was completely unassailable. The construction was in conformity with the building permit and the town planning regulations down to the smallest detail. But this legal disruption lasted two years all the same, since our charming neighbor, not content to see her suit dismissed at the court of first instance, filed an appeal, only to find herself condemned to pay us a significant fine for abuse of process.

I can assure you that during these two years our minds were never at ease. Although we knew that we were in the right, we couldn't help but imagine the worst. Court decisions are not always predictable. If we received a demolition order, it would mean financial ruin and living in the street for the rest of our lives!

But well before this happy conclusion, our second general contractor was unceremoniously fired from his company (I wonder why!), when the house had only just recently been sealed from the elements. Our budget could not be indefinitely extended, it was impossible to hire a new general contractor. We thus faced a dilemma: go to court to make the contracting company honor its commitments, which entailed bringing by experts to observe the status of the construction and all the defects, then wait probably several years for a court decision before the construction site could get started again, or finish the house ourselves. Disgusted with legal proceedings and impatient to move in, we quickly opted for the second solution. Our construction site thus turned into a DIY project in spite of ourselves. From this moment on, all our nights and weekends were spent with hammers, saws, screwdrivers, and paintbrushes in hand.

But the jinx didn't let up and our dump of a rental started to cause us major frustrations. Since we moved in, we struggled against the proliferation of mold in every room, against the rain that dripped in along the woodwork, the ants and the slugs that invaded the kitchen... The owner was not cooperative and we had other fish to fry than to harass her, so we had to grit our teeth and let it go. But all at once, in the space of a few weeks, a series of disasters occurred: both the electrical installation and the gas-fired boiler died on us, which left us with no heat or hot water for three weeks in the middle of December, an old dead tree began to collapse on top of the roof, a storm uprooted two 15-meter pine trees in the garden, the wastewater leach field clogged up, which made it impossible to flush the toilets, the internet connection would cut off for several days each week...and so on. The owner was begrudgingly forced to take measures, and we soon found ourselves having to put up with works in our temporary accommodations. The horror. Complete refurbishment of the roof, insulation, repair of the electrical installation, installation of a mechanically controlled ventilation system, clearing of terrain...

But we took everything philosophically. We didn't even keep track of the delay in our construction anymore. The main thing was that things continued to move forward, at least a little bit. Step by step, the house ended up becoming almost livable a few months after my burnout, and four years after we filed the first application for a building permit! There were hundreds of things to still finalize, but nevertheless in March 2020 we decided to move in – and it was a good thing we did, because two days later, the government declared the first COVID-19 lockdown. Paradoxically, this lockdown was one of the happiest periods of our lives.

It has to be acknowledged: these four years were a real hell. Nevertheless, all the stress and mental overload that I had to put up with is not enough to explain what triggered my burnout. It's true that my resiliency was necessarily affected during this period, but when we fight for something we dream of, something we've chosen, our resources are tremendous. Some people live through things infinitely more grueling and don't collapse under the weight.

It was thus necessary to keep searching for the underlying causes of my burnout. My psychologist asked me to reflect on conflicts of values that I've dealt with and this time, it was the working world that I had to delve into.

5 Alienation at work

I'm not going to inflict on you a complete account of my career and all the aggravations that put stomach in knots. It wouldn't even be very interesting, since we all experience difficulties at work. So I have selected for you a compendium of topics and vignettes that I find particularly representative of the mechanisms of alienation to which we find ourselves more or less exposed.

To start out gently, I will speak to you about a rather surprising topic: clothing. It's a subject that is possibly of no great seriousness, but which is nonetheless revealing about the level of alienation to which we are commonly subjected without even realizing it! It is something that has followed me throughout my career, in all the different companies that I've worked for.

My first shock came in 2004. I had just become manager of a small team of four people, and we had the opportunity to take on a young trainee technician. Like many young people of his age, he was not a big fan of doing laundry or ironing and he regularly arrived at work with completely crumpled t-shirts.

As you know, in the business world, there are lots of implicit codes, and manner of dress is one of them. Even if things have evolved significantly in recent years, it is always in good taste to dress "smart" without necessarily being stuffy. Apparently, the problem is that not everyone has the same perception of what it means to dress "smart." The "suit and tie" are almost no longer used nowadays, but an (ironed) dress shirt and long trousers are still the standard in many businesses. One day, my superior cornered me in a hallway and told me that I absolutely had to speak with my trainee to make him understand that an "effort to dress nice" was expected of him – at the very least, he needed to iron his shirts. "You're his manager, it's your job to instill in him the codes of the working world."

Needless to say, I was very uncomfortable. I had no desire to go make this hurtful remark to this young man who in all other respects did excellent work and only deserved encouragement. But on the other hand, it was necessary to make him aware of this famous dress code that could cause him problems in the future.

I didn't want to be hasty and mulled over the problem for several days, until a discussion over coffee with a colleague finally shed some light on the situation. He told me, "You know, when people have a different perception on a subject, the only thing that matters is what the law says." It so happens that this colleague had been staff representative for several years, so he had some instincts in this sense. He helped me dig up the company's internal regulations and the relevant passages of the Labor Code on the dress code. The internal regulation did not mention any dress requirements at all, and with good reason, as that would be totally illegal, since Article L1121-1 of the Labor Code is unequivocal about this: "Nobody shall impose on the rights of persons or on individual and collective freedoms any restrictions that are not justified by the nature of the task and proportionate to the desired aim." Basically, employers simply do not have the right to impose the least dress requirement on their employees outside of "personal protective equipment" or "presentable clothing" during a client visit for example, or if they have a stand at the trade fair or at the company's reception desk, etc.

Therefore, my superior was in fact asking me to do something illegal. Even worse, making this type of remark to one of my subordinates could constitute harassment!

I hurried to share my findings with my superior, who had a very cowardly reaction. "Oh yes, you're referring to his wrinkled t-shirts. Well, I was just saying that in case you could slip him a word as a friend, obviously we couldn't make the comment to him formally."

Unfortunately, this experience came in handy for me time and again over the course of my career. Two years later, I had to defend one of my best designers, whom management wanted to lay off after he showed up at a staff meeting without wearing the shirt with the company's colors. Ten years later, a young colleague committed the outrage of showing up in the design office in "capri pants" as a way of surviving a breakdown in the A/C. The old hags of the office next door were shocked to see his hairy calves and had a word with management. And I can't even speak about the young ladies that I had on my team who had to put up with regular comments, including from management, about their outfits that were too revealing or too attention-grabbing, about their hairstyles, their piercings, their tattoos...I saw these young women stoically put up with these remarks that they would have never tolerated in their personal lives. But when it happens at work, we have the impression that it's our job and our recognition that are at stake, and so we automatically push back the limits of what we're willing to accept.

Oh yes, our manner of dress and, more broadly, physical appearance are areas that we take too lightly. They often give rise to teasing among colleagues, but when it's a question of orders coming from the hierarchy, it's a major act of violence. The individual feels deprived of their right to their own personality. We tell them to fit into a mold, to undergo alienation.

I was never a victim of such orders as a staff member (that would be a sight to see!), but I experienced these injustices in full force as a manager who had to defend his teams. At these times, I felt misunderstood and brutalized by unscrupulous directors who were ignorant of the law. Even in my regard, they tried to alienate me in the role of someone who must embody and defend a certain vision of the ideal appearance of an employee.

The following topic has to do with the strategic bad faith of certain companies.

When you join a company, you are generally happy to adopt its state of mind, to identify with this image that attracted us in the first place. But when you find out that this company misbehaves in the marketplace, it can be devastating, you can feel used and betrayed.

At the start of my career, I worked for a dozen years in the automobile industry. It's a hard, uncompromising field, but also exhilarating, when you're a young engineer who's passionate about technology. I was happy to help personal transport advance toward solutions that were more effective, more pleasant, and more respectful of the environment.

But contact with this world threw cold water on my vision. I came to realize that most of my colleagues were more passionate about "heavy machinery" than they were about change and innovation. They were eager to burn gasoline and burn rubber when the weekend arrived, and any vehicle of less than 100 horsepower didn't even merit their attention. This mentality was largely encouraged by management, which paid for courses on the racetrack and big, polluting company cars for their most deserving employees.

I felt like a sheep among a pack of wolves. With my more environmentalist sensibility, I wasn't interested in opening up during our coffee break. When I arrived by bike one morning, my colleagues looked at me with a pitying glance. "You should have told me that your car was in the shop, I would have come to pick you up!"

But the mindset was beginning to evolve, we started to talk of the end of oil, atmospheric pollution was at the center of the political debate and certain scientists were even advancing the crazy idea that the climate was changing. So I quietly told myself, "That's it, the automobile world is going to undergo a change, we don't have a choice," and I was impatient to finally make my contribution to this change. Several colleagues around me started to open their mouth, criticizing the cult of the big gas guzzler, and started coming by bus or by train. In the lab, we were testing hybrid cars to measure reductions in fuel consumption, we were following the technological evolution of batteries, and the marketing department struggled to understand the changes in our society.

I will never forget the International Motor Show in Frankfurt in 2007, the year of the so-called wake-up call of the automobile world. All the booths were painted green, there were trees and planets on all the logos, there was competition to see whose cars would post the lowest fuel consumption. But when I saw that even the manufacturers of big SUVs were playing up their environmental efforts, I quickly understood the turn that things were going to take: we were entering a major era of "green washing" (the art of presenting a product as environmentally friendly when it isn't particularly so).

The management of my company did not hesitate to deploy this new vision. It was absolutely necessary to ride this environmentalist trend, but all while changing as little as possible in our industry, as a way to extract the most profit from our past investments. All of the sudden, it was a bonanza: products that we had been making for 15 years now had a thousand new virtues. It was enough to change one detail, to add one anecdotal function and we could boast of leading a green revolution. It was at this time that the actions that would later lead to the famous Dieselgate were committed: certain manufacturers tampered with the programming of the engine control unit to make it capable of detecting the moment when the car is undergoing emissions testing. At that point, the unit would change the engine settings in order to receive a good score for emissions and fuel consumption...but just during the test. Meanwhile, on the road, these cars would release ever more black clouds upon start-up.

On our side, we worked on small innovations like "Stop-and-Start," which consists of cutting off the motor automatically when it's not being used. Nowadays that seems ludicrous in light of the massive environmental challenges that we have to face. For my part, this was a long period of alienation, where I honestly wasn't free to propose the innovations that seemed the most promising to me, although it was a large part of the mission that I was hired for. In front of our clients, I had to defend our arguments, even if I knew that they were bogus. They asked me to communicate the company line. Project management was also a major source of frustration, since I could see that we were wasting our R&D budgets on topics that really didn't contribute toward a better future for the planet. When I spoke up with management to defend my ideas, they explained to me that the priority was to work on the products most likely to quickly generate the most revenue, that we weren't philanthropists responsible for saving the world. We even had some projects that only existed to drain public finances. We knew perfectly well that they would never lead to anything, the aim was rather to make them last as long as possible. As a result, every year I spent ages drawing up the paperwork for the "research tax credit" in order to extract money from the government.

The third topic has to do with the cowardice of management. Those situations where management asks you to do their dirty work for them. Unfortunately, I could cite numerous examples, but I will only subject you to one of them that particularly traumatized me.

It had been a few months since I started with a new company as head of a design office of seven to eight people. We were growing and had just recruited two young technicians for a fixed-term contract of six months. One of them was reaching the end of his contract and as the work was going well, we needed to reinforce the team on a long-term basis, so we were thinking about offering him an open-ended contract.

My superior updated the budget and the business plan and went up to see the Managing Director in order to get permission for this hire. It was all logical and well-supported, so the Managing Director gave his blessing, though not without first checking the numbers at great length. The young man had a number of vacation days to use up before the end of his contract, so he had planned on taking off for the next two weeks. My superior asked me to quickly let him know that we planned on offering him an open-ended contract upon his return, lest he take advantage of these two weeks to look for work elsewhere. I thus had the pleasure of giving him this good news one-on-one in a room, when giving him his job performance review. He was overjoyed and left for vacation with a smile.

It goes without saying, the inevitable happened: one of the markets served by our company had been slowing down for several months and, when the moment came to tally the financial results of the quarter, it was a big hullabaloo. Management was shocked to see results that were below the projections. They put in place immediate financial restrictions and a freeze on new hires. My superior defended our young technician tooth and nail, highlighting the fact that my design office was situated in a booming market that helped restore our revenue and so it was necessary to bolster our team. But it was no use, the Managing Director categorically refused to sign the contract. I also raised the issue with human resources, noting that our position was legally dubious, since the message they had asked me to deliver to our young man was nothing more or less than a hiring notification that we couldn't retract. The director of human resources cynically told me that we were at no risk, since he had no means to prove it. In passing, she remarked to me that I myself was at the end of my probation period and she didn't like my attitude!

Announcing this bad news to my technician when he returned from leave was one of the most difficult moments of my career. It gives me a knot in my stomach even today. I was always in the habit of doing the difficult and unpleasant things at work. Bearing bad news or raising complaints was part of a manager's daily job. But in this case, it was different: management had betrayed us and I was forced to deliver a message that wasn't mine. I would have appreciated it if the Managing Director had borne the consequences of his decision by coming himself to communicate it to this person, rather than using me to do his dirty work.

Then how can I discuss managerial failures without mentioning the issue of technical incompetence? It is perhaps the most instructive scourge of the business world, which has not ceased to amaze me since the beginning of my career and which causes significant damage to company efficiency and the relationship that employees have with their work. Not only are there relatively few managers who have real managerial skills, but the overwhelming majority of them are not even experts in the technical domain in which they work either! Unlike the Japanese model where an employee must start "at the bottom of the ladder" (what a horrible expression!) and must climb the ladder by proving their worth, our Western model follows the opposite logic: the manager is decreed from on high and is instantaneously hoisted up on a pedestal. It's a matter of title, and sometimes even a reward. So we have to trust them before they even prove themselves. He's the boss, he's the one who takes major decisions, and yet we can't even expect that he's mastered the substance of what he's managing. That really takes the cake!

In my case, when I became a manager, I had already practiced my profession of product designer for six years. Even if I was far from mastering everything, I had acquired a certain experience and I was happy to share it and put it to use in taking decisions that could have a more direct effect on the quality of the products we were putting on the market. But from the very first days since I took on this position, my superior told me: "Go to the IT department and ask them for a laptop, since you will need it to conduct meetings...Then tell them to terminate your access to the CAD (computer-aided design) software. You won't be needing it anymore."

Excuse me? How was that possible? Do we ask a stonemason to give up his boots because he becomes a foreman? Do we ask a baker to no longer touch flour because he hires some employees? How could I direct, train and evaluate my team if I distance myself from my profession? For this reason, I fought tooth and nail to keep my CAD licenses, and with hindsight, I am glad I did. It wasn't easy though. In all the companies where I worked, I had to struggle against this aberration. They refused to train me on new tools, so I trained myself all on my own, they didn't want to give me a high-performing work station, so I ran these huge programs in reduced functionality mode on my poor office PC...but I always kept going and fortunately, I did so without becoming one of those managers who manage nothing but hot air, who put pressure on their subordinates without providing them with the means or the instructions that they need, who fill out annual evaluations by guesswork, without having a precise idea of what these expected skills really consist of.

Of course, when you manage a team of designers, you're only rarely called upon to carry out concrete tasks like 3D modeling, drafting, choice of materials, or mechanical stress calculations. But in any case, you still have to evaluate the results and give instructions in order to make adjustments. In the end, it remains a design step in its own right, with more delegation of tasks but with just as weighty a responsibility for the final result. In other words, the designer and his manager practice the same basic profession, it's only the position that changes! Since I kept up my mastery of design tools, I never had to bother my staff to extract product images in order to illustrate a presentation, tap them on the shoulder to open a 3D model sent by a client, pester them to outline a change proposal or to print out designs to show to a supplier. I was always able to train young recruits on the tools and procedures, help them out when they were having trouble with a technical choice or a material obstacle, etc.

I'm proud of having maintained this integrity, this fundamental link with the underlying know-how of my profession. On the other hand, I have been able to observe on a daily basis to what extent my fellow managers or my superiors in the hierarchy have succumbed and have lost this link, to the point that they are no longer at all capable of making technical decisions. When it was a question of deciding the fate of a product, looking for ways to improve it, to resolve a defect, to improve our tools or our working methods, they didn't have a clue. Nobody knew what to do and, very often it ended in convoluted, unfortunate decisions, such as calling upon external firms that were even more removed from the topic.

Having to make my career within this environment where incompetence was normalized and accepted wore me out in a profound way. Very often I played the role – in spite of myself – of the guy they call for help in desperate situations, as the only one capable of understanding certain technical problems. But the recognition and satisfaction that should have been my due turned out to be very slim, as I found myself bogged down in a quagmire that

I hadn't created and which I had very little power to improve.

Let's move on to the fifth topic of alienation: the "corporate culture." It's very fashionable lately and as surprising as it may seem, it's one of the biggest sources of alienation in our daily life. There's nothing mean-spirited about it at all, but it creates fertile ground for burnout to appear, since we expect employees to adhere to common values, that they acquire certain qualities and certain pre-established behaviors, that they slip into the role of ideal employee, that they perfectly embody the company's personality and not their own.

But it's no big deal, we could almost call that "positive alienation." After all, we're only trying to help people become better, no? And in the end, employees are only alienated during the time that they're at work, free to become themselves again when they go back home.

But let's think about it for second: is it written in the work contract or in the Labor Code that employees are required to conform to a corporate culture? That they must embody the values we impose on them? That they have to do everything to spread friendliness and good cheer around them? Of course not! Even if they are always well-intentioned, these practices emerge from an abusive interpretation of the relationship between employer and employee. Generally speaking, anything that involves dominance and control has no role in a professional relationship. Employees don't "belong" to their employer and they don't have the duty to be actors.

And conversely, employees shouldn't think that the company owes them perfect happiness. It's not a mother that's supposed to meet all their needs. The work contract doesn't stipulate that the company has the obligation to guarantee a better life for its employees, an ever-increasing salary, an idyllic working environment, or that it needs to protect them from any disappointment or misfortune.

A work contract is nothing more than an exchange of services, not a relationship of submission and domination. So why not just stick to that and forget about the rest?

Put yourself in the shoes of an employee drowning in work who struggles every day to make ends meet, stay focused on his targets to ensure the future and prosperity of the shop. He can't manage to do everything; he has to limit himself to the most urgent tasks and extend his working hours. And one day, we come to him and simperingly ask him to participate in a half-day reflection on the values of the company: "This is more important than everything else, you understand, it's what defines our identity." And several weeks later, it's a two-day seminar to "reinforce team cohesion." Then a one-day retreat on the "company mission." Then a workshop to organize the "company get-together," etc.

Giving contradictory orders is a violent act. Here, on the one hand, "You have to work hard and use your days well in order to reach the objectives of your assignment." On the other hand, "Come with us, free up your time to do some things that have nothing to do with your duties, even if it will put you in greater difficulty for all the rest."

More generally, is it really necessary to worry about well-being at work? It's a question of perception. Some people may feel content to find a "big family" at work, but for other people, it might seem like an unjustified requirement if they feel forced to get along with people that they wouldn't have chosen as friends of their own accord.

If affinities and common values must emerge between people, this has to be a natural process, we can't dictate their feelings. We need to let things happen on their own.

I think that trying to force well-being is to pick the wrong battle, since above all else, practicing our profession is what will cause us to flourish and not the surrounding conditions on their own, even if they contribute a little bit. So no, well-being at work doesn't mean redecorating the offices and putting in a foosball table in the break room. Real well-being is when people can do their job calmly and effectively, nothing more.

No, we don't create motivation at work – that is something simply induced by the conditions of the work contract, it can't be infinitely extended. Trying to develop an attractive company culture or to convince employees that "the company is a big family" are on the whole counterproductive and even destructive mechanisms.

For companies that bemoan an epidemic of burnout, the solution is easy: stop all high-handedness with their employees, stop the orders, trust them, stop policing them, ease up on everything that makes their daily lives more complicated. We have to leave them free to develop their tools and environment, we have to give them a certain flexibility over their hours and their days off, and allow them the option to work from home as often as possible.

By removing some of the friction between professional life and personal life, we allow everyone to disalienate themselves more easily when they go home. We encourage their brains to construct solid reference points to distinguish between those things that relate to the role they must play at work and those things that relate to "real life," where our inner self regains the upper hand.

A common mistake is to try to establish material markers to help us distinguish these moments of transition from one role to another: I get in the car to go home, so I stop thinking about work and turn off my professional cell phone. OK, why not, it's radical. Except that the real boundaries are psychological and associating them with material markers is a dangerous habit that can lead to deceiving the brain and fueling confusion.

I think we can all agree that if your boss calls you on the weekend, it's just intolerable. But if that call is to let you know that he won't be able to pick you up at the planned place on Monday morning to go visit the client, then it has nothing to do with interfering with your private life, it's just basic good manners. So be careful not to confuse "right to disconnect" and "duty to disconnect"!

I find it infinitely healthier to leave your phone on, even if you berate your boss without mercy if he abuses it, because depriving yourself of the possibility of being reached in case of real necessity will not make your life any easier either.

The example of teleworking is even more glaring: many people completely sink in this context that deprives them of the small material markers they were used to. Suddenly, it's total blur. Can I allow myself to get up from my desk to go get a coffee? To open the door to the delivery man? To take care of my sick child? To take time off for a medical appointment? We can see that here, the usual logic of disconnection guided by material markers no longer makes any sense. Your only chance is to exercise your brain to spot at every moment if you are working for yourself or for your employer, if you are supposed to be available for work or for real life, and to regularly assess the amount of energy and/or time you allocate to each role. It is also this awareness and this alone that will allow you to voluntarily leave one role to seek refuge in the other in order to give yourself beneficial breaks.

It is not because you are at home, phone turned off, that your mind is not at risk of being overwhelmed by the troubles of work, but only because you have consciously decided to fully dedicate yourself to your personal life at that moment. This liberating mechanism can only be psychological, not material.

Furthermore, I've always been surprised at that type of anxiety felt by company management that is persuaded that it is absolutely necessary to keep people under their thumb out of fear that they will refuse to obey or will work less. It's completely absurd. Personally, I can't think of a single example of an employee who one day would refuse to do what's asked of him. Sometimes, there may be misunderstandings or reluctance, but outright insubordination is extremely rare. And with good reason: employees are there of their own free will, and if they remain there, it's because the conditions of their work contract are satisfactory for them. The day that's no longer the case, they will leave, and that's an entirely healthy mechanism.

As for keeping people under your thumb in order to try to get them to work more, that just doesn't work: we all have a certain amount of energy at our disposal. Even if we're all able to make an extra effort when necessary, that can't be a permanent state of affairs. What's more, this extra effort always comes at the expense of other efforts that we let up on, whether in our personal or our professional lives, and in the medium term we have to pay for the consequences on our effectiveness. Thus, the only real leverage the company has is to get people to appreciate their job, so that it inspires them to dedicate a greater part of that limited energy that they have.

I've spent 24 years fulminating against people who don't do a damn thing at work: you know, the people who are always in a meeting or behind a Powerpoint, monitoring indicators they don't understand, giving lessons and doling out criticism, but who don't produce anything solid themselves. I'm sure you can see I know what I'm talking about, the working world is plagued with these people. So is it these people who were right all along? In the end, they protect themselves pretty well. By not getting too involved, they don't run the risk of alienation. Is it necessary to be a slacker with a cushy job to preserve oneself? I'm not sure, but I can observe that many people seem to have chosen this route and they are no more worse off for it.

On the other hand, when we're passionate about our work, when we're hard-working and eager to share in our colleague's efforts, we soon find ourselves over-involved and in a dangerous spiral: the more effective and productive we are, the more useful we are to others and the more they seek us out.

But in the end, it's not so much this that's the problem, since, as there's only 24 hours in a day and our energy is not inexhaustible, our efforts tend to self-regulate on their own. The problem then are all those things in daily life that prevent us from doing our work. Those over-rigid and absurd procedures, those days spent chasing down elusive bosses to have them sign a piece of paper, budgets and expenses to justify the least detail, unsuitable IT tools, invented and secured by people who will never use them, that maddeningly slow internet connection, the phone plan that you have to watch to the last cent, those endless, useless meetings that you can't get out of.

In my previous position, it was required for all managers to input their team's daily schedule into four different tools. This task alone took us an hour and a half each day! And, of course, my repeated and urgent requests to the leadership to consolidate these four tools into one were never successful. How can such absurdity reach such heights without anyone being able to change it?

But then again, that's nothing out of the ordinary, everybody goes through that on a daily basis without suffering burnout. The frustrations begin when we see slogans posted on the wall that encourage us to "keep it simple," "avoid waste," "be effective," to work "lean" and with "ongoing improvement."

When we organize seminars to collect good ideas that are likely to really change things. Finally, we'll be able to get rid of all these daily hassles! Then little by little, we suffer disappointment and frustration, since we realize that all these efforts toward change that are put in place are later scuttled and derailed by these same people who encourage us to propose them. New tools and new procedures replace the old ones, and they turn out to be even worse, even less flexible. We find ourselves subjected to even more control and oversight. The more we advance, the less people work and the more they go in circles, lost in navel-gazing.

That's where alienation begins, with having to go along with nonsense and show forced enthusiasm, when we only ever wanted to be able to do our job correctly.

The worst thing about this is that the operation of companies doesn't seem to rest on any positive feedback loop. To the contrary, they are in a permanent state of collapse that needs constant rebuilding, all while expending an insane amount of energy. Incidentally, that's why many businesses have a department dedicated to "ongoing improvement." It's an admission of failure in and of itself, since there would be no need for it if the company's mechanisms were able to improve themselves on their own, along the lines of the evolution of species in nature. In fact, everything unfolds as if "sinecured slackers" were in power, regardless of their position in the hierarchy, perhaps simply because they have more time to get their point across than the hard workers busting their hump.

Over the course of my career, I've had the good fortune to attain some real professional success, putting on the market products that users have adored and acclaimed. On these occasions, I expected that all the members of the company – hierarchy, colleagues, experts, trainers – would come seek me out to try to draw some lessons about what worked well and to learn from the mistakes that I made. I expected a certain form of Darwinism that would have successful projects serve as an example to help the organization's tools evolve. But every time, the opposite phenomenon occurred: my team and me personally became suspect, as if they suspected us of having infringed on the procedures and of having taken shameful liberties in order to succeed where the normal course of things usually led to mediocrity or failure.

There are many works on organizational failures in the business world and how to avoid them, so I won't enlarge on the subject. But without a doubt, this situation was a potent catalyst for my breakdown.

6 Cultural alienation

Finally, I would like to describe for you another type of alienation that weighed heavily in my case: cultural alienation. It's certainly not by chance that the number of victims of burnout exploded in recent decades, while the business world was globalizing.

How is it that company managers could have imagined for a single second that we could calmly do business while ignoring cultural differences and geopolitical constraints? That we could put together multinational teams and let them muddle through while disregarding their conflicts of interest? Having witnessed all this from the front row, I can affirm that not only have outsourcing and globalization been a disaster for France's industrial base, they have also had devastating consequences for the mental health of many employees. In fact, we often find ourselves very easily caught between orders from management that thinks "all you have to do is…" and the reality on the ground that is a constant struggle.

For my part, I've always practiced my profession in a globalized context ever since my very first job, when I worked for a Malaysian industrial group, then in the automobile industry where I interfaced on a daily basis with teams located in Poland, South Korea and India, and finally in a multimarket industry where my teams and my contacts were scattered across France, China, India, the US, Mexico, Sweden and Finland. Accordingly, during these 24 years, multicultural interactions have been part of my daily job.

Even if I've always appreciated interaction with other cultures, I've often been flabbergasted by the naivety of my hierarchy, or even by their cynicism when faced with the difficulties that this multicultural context would cause. When I sought more resources to reinforce my team, nine times out of ten the response of my superiors would be "OK no problem, I'll give you three Indians" or "We'll put this project in China." Of course, on paper, it's practical and it costs much less. In real life, however, it ends up totally dooming a project. But nobody wants to hear that, it's a big taboo, it's politically incorrect to say it, because that would seem to imply that "these people are inferior." No, they are not inferior at all, they are just far away, they have a very different way of doing things and very different interests that are sometimes even completely opposed to ours.

In such situations, there are always only two possible outcomes: either we had to oversee the project very closely so that it would turn out like we hoped, in which case, we ended up spending much more time and energy on it than if we had carried it out ourselves, or we had to accept that the outcome would not be what we expected, and that was often very disappointing.

International interactions are absolutely necessary, no country can live in isolation. But it is necessary to be clear-headed about this: there are some barriers that we simply can't overcome. Let me describe a few of them.

One of them is clearly the fact of working with countries with significant material difficulties, like India. The cultural differences are already massive with this country, but however much we organize in order to surmount them, the fact will remain that we are dealing with a country where nothing works correctly. Both the electricity and the Internet go out several times a day, transportation is slow and unpredictable, corruption is everywhere, institutions are apathetic, and there are many serious health problems. In the end, everything goes more slowly and even the idea of planning doesn't work amid so many disruptions.

But of course, these realities are not understood by a French hierarchy that is focused – and rightly so – on the outcome, but which doesn't take seriously the amusing mishaps we tell them about and which never learns the proper lesson from this.

In reality, you'd have to be naïve or blind to cling to the least notion of performance in a country where people have daily worries much more serious than hitting the professional objectives we've set for them!

The second example is the cultural chasm with China, which is much deeper than we first imagine. Personally, it has taken me years to understand the extent of the repercussions involved in working with the inhabitants of a dictatorial regime.

My eureka moment occurred one morning when I was walking on a sidewalk in Shanghai on my way to visit our local factory. Bikes and scooters flowed by in an endless stream and all of a sudden, an old woman took a violent fall with her scooter about a dozen meters ahead of me.

At first, I remained paralyzed, not knowing whether I should intervene or not. There were a lot of people on the sidewalk, including a police officer, who subtly looked away, but nobody stopped, neither from among the pedestrians nor among the other motorcyclists, who pushed the body of this poor woman away with their feet in order to clear the way. I ultimately reached where she was and I couldn't not come to her aid: check if she was injured and help pick up her scooter in order to put it on the side of the street. She didn't understand English and I didn't speak Chinese, so our conversation was limited to a few stammered words. I could see that she was very upset, doubtlessly ashamed that only a foreigner had reacted. She quickly limped away, pushing her scooter with her. I was shocked. When I arrived at the office, I hastened to relate my misadventure to my Chinese colleagues and they all had the same reaction: "You are completely crazy to have intervened, you could have had some major problems! The police could have picked you up, and even the victim could have filed a complaint against you, accusing you of being responsible in order to extort damages from you."

This experience was a major epiphany for me. As someone who naively thought that mutual assistance and aid are universal values, I found myself confronted with a civilization where their behavior was totally distorted by this way of life under regime oppression. Above all, don't take risks, don't make waves, it's a question of survival, in a context where any member of the regime has the right to interpret the facts as they deem fit, with all the consequences you might imagine.

Afterwards, I found this same behavior on several levels in professional relationships, it became blindingly obvious. People who buried their heads in the sand instead of helping one another, the paranoia of the hierarchy, things done on the sly, incidents they would sweep under the rug in order to avoid problems, surveillance by party members present in every company, the subtly concealed corruption...

I've told this incident to my hierarchy in France time and again, but they never seemed to grasp what lessons we could learn from it. In what way should that have called into question our outsourcing to that country? Yet again, I found myself in the role of someone who had to pretend that it was no big deal, all the while every day I could see examples of serious dysfunctions and their disastrous consequences for our company: suppliers who scammed us on the quality of the raw materials while we couldn't say anything, local competitors who robbed us while being backed by the regime, clients who took advantage of our goodwill by having us develop products that they passed along to their fellow countrymen, the inability of people to recognize and admit their mistakes or risk "losing face," etc.

But cultural alienation isn't only caused by coming face-to-face with the practices of other cultures. Sometimes, it's our own culture that drives us to destruction. In France, we are encouraged from a very young age to give it our all in every field without necessarily understanding the point right away: at school, in sports, in extracurricular activities, then in higher education. We are convinced that it is only by making huge efforts that we can attain happiness, that it's a sort of heroic sacrifice. Then when we reach adulthood, we continue to perpetuate this behavior at work. Now I realize to what extent I was mired in this trap of overinvestment. Not only did my work engross me, but everyone around me encouraged me to work my fingers to the bone: my hierarchy, my family, my friends...This culture of heroism is a component of our civilization that we can't escape. But when work loses its meaning, the downward spiral into alienation is only all the more intense.

Finally, the third example involves taking into account the regulatory and normative differences between countries. Here it's not only a question of cultural divergences, but outright conflicts of interest.

Every year at Christmastime, consumer organizations publish alarmist reports about toys from China that turn out to be dangerous for children: potentially toxic materials, pieces that come off and could be swallowed...Why the hell do we allow the importation of products that don't meet the standards we impose on ourselves for products made in France? By the same token, why do we find in the supermarkets vegetables that come from countries where laws on the use of pesticides are lax or non-existent, while our own farmers are subjected to drastic requirements?

Well, it's exactly the same thing in the industrial world: when we design a product in France, we impose on ourselves very onerous quality standards, both on the performance of the products and on the methods for developing and manufacturing them. In and of itself, it's a good thing, since we strive to only produce "good" products from the point of view of the consumer – something I've always fiercely defended. But these standards have the effect of considerably increasing the costs and the time to market. So why not follow through and protect ourselves from competition from these "bad" products that don't respect these standards?

I can't count the number of times that a client has waved under my nose a competing product from China and said, "Look, it's half as expensive as your product, it does the same thing, and it's been on the market for three months." And every time I respond, "Yes, we're quite aware of this product, but it doesn't pass the tests imposed by the standards of your sector: in two years, it will become brittle from the effect of the sun, it contains prohibited plastic materials, and it is highly flammable." But they couldn't care less. In case of a problem, they would only have to take action against the unscrupulous supplier, who themselves always had a way out under their sleeve.

In this type of situation, the real loser is the end user of the product.

In fact, it's a real social choice that nobody has ever solved: do we want a French marketplace invaded with cheap but lousy products, or should we limit it to those that meet the minimum level of expectation that we impose on ourselves, even if they end up being more expensive?

What I'm decrying here is the violence of a globalized system that on the one hand, imposes drastic local constraints on manufacturers, but on the other hand, doesn't apply any arbitrage on the market. Do you think that China, for its part, refrains from banning products it doesn't like from its market?

We the French have spent generations building a culture and systems of quality that places us among the most capable of creating "good" products. Our industry demonstrates it every day. But why don't we do anything to protect ourselves from "bad" products that enter into direct competition with our own? Is it always necessary to leave it to commercial freedom and the self-regulation of the market? Do we really have to let the consumer decide? Are they even able to? Won't they just foolishly get hoodwinked by a lower price and seductive appearance?

In reality, the Darwinism of the market is unrelenting: bad products always stop selling in the end, to the benefit of good products. But the problem is that this operates over the long term and, in the meanwhile, we don't come out unscathed. That's precisely why globalization has totally stripped France of its industrial base. Now at this point, we've reached the stage where Darwinism has done its work: nobody wants Made in China, we want our products to be practical, well-designed, durable and repairable. We also wish to consume locally and no longer depend on potentially hostile powers. But the damage has been done, it will take major efforts to rebuild our industrial base.

With regards to product design, the naivety of our country and of Europe in the face of globalization has been a major source of difficulties and frustrations. I suffered from this every day. The efforts of me and my team to make our products ever better were systematically undermined by the short-term vision of the market, which preferred botched products from low-cost areas. And when, after a certain length of time, history proved us right, it was already too late, opportunity had passed us by.

7   Conclusion: It's nobody's fault

There you have it. It's because of all the above that I suffered a burnout. Does that surprise you?

To be sure, the mounting frustrations, stress and overload had a great deal to do with it, but the real underlying cause that left me without a chance was that I allowed myself to be confined for so long in roles that were in contradiction with my identity and my convictions.

All the urgings of my loved ones and doctors would not have been able to change anything. "You've got to slow down, you're doing too much, learn to say no, force yourself to delegate..." All of that was irrelevant, it wasn't the root of the problem. Yes indeed, being under pressure, stressed and swamped by mental overload is not a good thing. These are aggravating conditions that accelerate the onset of burnout by wearing down our resistance.

But human beings are designed to forcefully resist stress and pressure. History has shown us time and again: when he fights to defend his own ideas, Man has the capacity to overcome the worst affronts. It's not the same thing when he's forced to fight for ideas that are not his own.

And with good reason, if there's something that we're vulnerable to, it's alienation! Evolution hasn't really prepared us for that. It's true that, since the dawn of time, techniques of manipulation have been part of Man's daily life: in the realms of politics, religion, commerce, love...But who could have foreseen that our civilization would enter into a period where being alienated is commonplace! Even worse, a daily necessity! After all, you have to work hard to earn your daily bread, life isn't a cakewalk, you have to make efforts and concessions. So sign the contract and follow the instructions. When the time comes, you'll go announce to your colleagues that they're fired, you know, all these people they told you to love and respect because "we're all part of a big family"!

Burnout is a misfortune all the more difficult to live through because "it's nobody's fault." At times, you feel like blaming the whole world. It would be so much easier to tell ourselves that the fault belongs to our employers who pushed us too hard or didn't protect us enough, but the reality is more complicated. When it comes down to it, nobody is forcing us to take on so radically these roles that destroy us. It's rather the result of a cascade of bad practices and cultural deviations. When we sign a work contract, we know perfectly well that we are going to work to satisfy the interest of other people and that this will often come at the expense of our own ideas and convictions. We know it's bad, but we accept it. And it's very difficult to draw the line between what's acceptable and what's not.

I don't adhere to a vision of society along the lines of Émile Zola, where the nice employees are oppressed by the mean bosses, nor do I hold the converse view, where the motivations of bosses are always justifiable in the face of employees who should mind their own business. I think that we would all get on much better if we simply stuck to carrying out the terms of the work contract, no more and no less: perform professional duties in exchange for a salary. I am convinced that everything that falls outside this framework is risky and rarely desirable.

I would like to end with a positive message for all those who face burnout in some way. Some ordeals are sometimes also real opportunities for change, that are likely to lead us to something better. I know, it's a little cliché to say it, but, in the case of a burnout, it's necessary to understand that we absolutely don't have a choice: healing must take place through change, quite simply because we are obliged to eradicate from our lives those things that have destroyed us. Continuity, the wish for everything to go back to the way it was before, cannot offer any effective path for healing if the root causes are still there.

As for me, after my major breakdown at the start of 2020, I remained on sick leave for four entire months and then gradually returned to work on a part-time basis for another four months before resuming full-time work. This return to work, although it was gradual, was painful and made me realize the absolute need to change my life. I suffered head on that notorious "psychological allergy" to the root causes that I described in Chapter 3. Every day was an ordeal that pulled me down. I had around me examples of colleagues who were also victims of burnout who had succumbed once and for all. I knew that, without a change in my life, I was running the risk of relapse and discouragement, only to find myself two or three years later shut up in my house with an inability to work.

As I had this planned career change up my sleeve to start on lutherie, the decision became a no-brainer. It was a leap into the unknown, nerve-wracking yet liberating. I was obviously not ready to embark on this career change so early, neither materially nor financially. But I realized that there would probably never be a better opportunity. In fact, it was my only chance to recover, since any other path would lead to a much worse situation. Accordingly, I left my job through a mutually-agreed termination with my employer, then I dedicated a year to professional development and building my company.

Two years after my burnout, I am now in the launch state of this new occupation and I am now discovering to what extent we're more effective and flourishing when we practice our profession in good conditions.

As for my symptoms, they have almost all disappeared.

Of course, I still have a way to go in order to get back into shape, you don't bounce back so quickly after two years of inactivity. But my body now responds again normally on its own accord, I almost never have to force myself anymore.

The famous "psychological allergy" to the causes that destroyed me is still present, but it is gradually diminishing. It's true, I still cannot put up with the high-handedness, the administrative and systemic aberrations, the orders of those who think they know better than me. Nor can I tolerate any form of alienation, of course. But in the end, I have learned to use this allergy as a "bad vibes detector" that has helped me to find my path in my new life without falling back into old habits. I've realized that the indispensable condition of my survival is to dedicate my energy only to things that are meaningful for me.

The most surprising thing of all, it's that from the moment that we decide to listen to ourselves, the planets seem to align. All the doors open. A wealth of favorable events and happy coincidences begin to happen, one after the other. The path to healing becomes a virtuous circle.

I am not well-versed in esoteric thought, but everything happens as if bad luck or providence are determined by our state of mind. However, it's not a question of perception, it's factual: I run into much fewer hassles now than four years ago. But maybe it's just the result of a chain reaction set off by my daily actions that I orient in a positive direction without even realizing it.

It could simply be that I'm becoming the protagonist of my life.

www.ingramcontent.com/pod-product-compliance
Lightning Source LLC
LaVergne TN
LVHW050913200726
843508LV00011B/2190